DIABETIC TYPE 2 GROCERY AND FOOD LIST

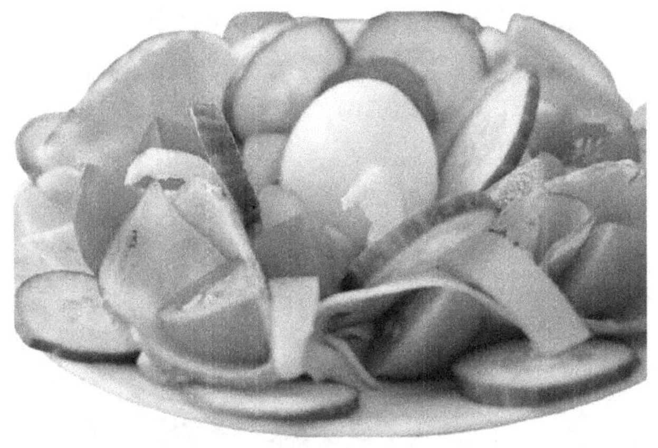

The Comprehensive Guide for Low Glycemic Index Nutrition with 30 Nutrient-Rich Recipes to Support Diabetes Reversal

Felicia O. Pace

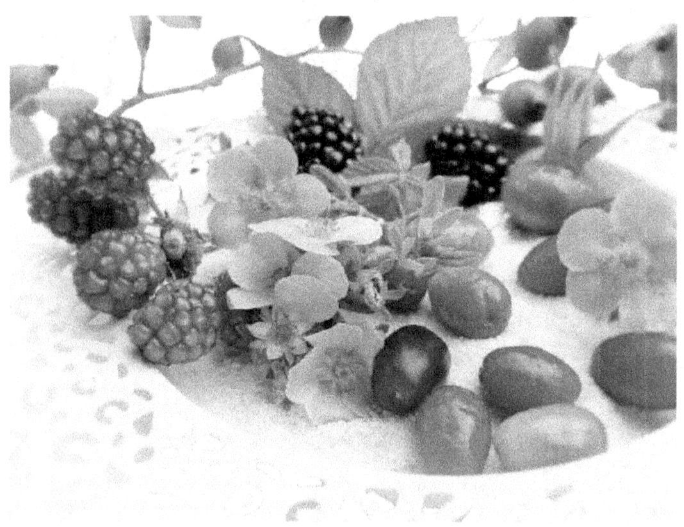

Table of Contents

LOW GLYCEMIC INDEX FOOD CHARTS: ORGANIZING INTRODUCTION 5

Why This Book? 6

Healthy diabetic-friendly Groceries List 8

fruits and vegetables 8

Lean Proteins 10

Fats and Oil 13

Legumes and Grains 15

Dairy Alternatives 19

Snacks 21

Sweetner and Condiments 24

Beverages 26

FOOD FOR CONVENIENT AND QUICK REFERENCE 29

Low GI Fruits 29

Low GI Vegetables 31

Low GI Legumes and Pulses 33

Low GI whole grains 35

Low GI Dairy and Dairy Alternatives 37

Low GI Nuts and Seed 39

Low GI proteins 41

Low GI fats and Oil 43

Low GI Snacks 45

Low GI Beverages...47

Low GI Seafood 49

Low GI Soup and Broths...51

Low GI Herbs and Spices 53

Low GI Sweeteners 55

Low GI Condiments and Sauces 57

Low GI Spreads and Dips...59

Low GI Dressing and Marinades 61

Low GI Baking and Cooking Ingredients...63

30 NUTRIENT-RICH LOW GI RECIPES...65

Breakfast 65

Lunch...69

Dinner...73

Snacks...77

Dessert 80

Smoothies 83

CONCLUSION...87

INTRODUCTION

In the journey towards managing and maintaining a healthy lifestyle with Type 2 Diabetes, the significance of a well-curated grocery and food list cannot be overstated. Living with Diabetes requires careful consideration of the foods we consume, as they play a pivotal role in regulating blood sugar levels, managing weight, and promoting overall well-being. This book is designed to empower individuals with Type 2 Diabetes with knowledge and practical insights into making informed choices while navigating the aisles of their local grocery store.

Understanding Diabetes and the Role of Diet
Type 2 Diabetes is a chronic condition characterized by insulin resistance, where the body's cells do not effectively use insulin, leading to elevated blood sugar levels. While genetics and other factors contribute to its development, lifestyle choices, including diet, play a crucial role. Proper nutrition becomes a cornerstone in managing Diabetes, aiding in glucose control and reducing the risk of complications.

This book aims to bridge the gap between nutritional science and everyday food choices, providing a comprehensive resource for individuals seeking clarity on what to include in their pantry and refrigerator. By understanding the impact of different foods on blood sugar levels, individuals can make mindful decisions that align with their health goals.

Creating a diabetic-friendly grocery list involves selecting foods that are nutrient-dense, low in added sugars, and have a favorable impact on glycemic response. *This book will explore various food categories of 300+ Recipes and 30 healthy and flavourful recipes* with offering detailed insights into fruits, vegetables, lean proteins, healthy fats, legumes, grains, dairy alternatives, snacks, sweeteners, condiments, and beverages. Each category will include essential items, complete with nutritional information, allowing for informed choices that cater to both taste preferences and health requirements.

Why This Book?

In a world inundated with information, it's easy to feel overwhelmed and confused about what to eat, especially for those managing Type 2 Diabetes. This book seeks to simplify the process, providing a clear roadmap for creating a diabetic-friendly kitchen. By incorporating a variety of nutritious foods and understanding their impact on blood sugar, individuals can confidently embrace a lifestyle that promotes health, well-being, and long-term Diabetes management.

Remember, this book is not a one-size-fits-all solution. It's a starting point—a foundation upon which individuals can build a personalized approach to nutrition. Consultation with healthcare professionals, including registered dietitians, is encouraged for tailored advice based on individual health needs.

Embark on this journey with the knowledge that food is not merely sustenance; it's a powerful tool in managing and thriving with Type 2 Diabetes. Let this guide be your companion in making informed, delicious, and health-conscious choices as you navigate the aisles and embrace a lifestyle that supports your well-being.

Healthy diabetic-friendly Groceries List

fruits and vegetables

1. Spinach:
Calories: 7 per cup
Sugar: 0.1 g

2. Broccoli:
Calories: 31 per cup
Sugar: 1.5 g

3. Blueberries:
Calories: 84 per cup
Sugar: 15 g

4. Avocado:
Calories: 234 per cup (sliced)
Sugar: 0.7 g

5. Strawberries:
Calories: 50 per cup
Sugar: 7.4 g

6. Cauliflower:
Calories: 25 per cup
Sugar: 2 g

7. Bell Peppers (Mixed Colors):
Calories: 46 per cup
Sugar: 6 g

8. Apples:
Calories: 95 per medium apple
Sugar: 19 g

9. Carrots:
Calories: 41 per cup
Sugar: 6 g

10. Raspberries:
Calories: 64 per cup
Sugar: 5.4 g

11. Kale:
Calories: 33 per cup
Sugar: 0 g

12. Oranges:
Calories: 62 per medium orange
Sugar: 12 g

13. Cucumbers:
Calories: 8 per half cup
Sugar: 1.9 g

14. Pears:
Calories: 101 per medium pear
Sugar: 17 g

15. Brussels Sprouts:
Calories: 38 per cup
Sugar: 2 g

16. Cherries:
Calories: 77 per cup
Sugar: 18 g

17. Zucchini:
Calories: 20 per cup
Sugar: 1.5 g

18. Grapes:
Calories: 104 per cup
Sugar: 23 g

19. Asparagus:
Calories: 27 per cup
Sugar: 1.9 g

20. Peaches:
Calories: 59 per medium peach
Sugar: 13 g

Lean Proteins

1. Chicken Breast (Skinless, Boneless):
Calories: 165 per 3.5 oz (cooked)
Sugar: 0 g

2. Turkey Breast (Skinless, Ground):
Calories: 135 per 3.5 oz (cooked)
Sugar: 0 g

3. Fish (Salmon):
Calories: 206 per 3.5 oz (cooked)
Sugar: 0 g

4. Tofu:
Calories: 144 per 3.5 oz (firm, cooked)
Sugar: 0.4 g

5. Shrimp:
Calories: 99 per 3.5 oz (cooked)
Sugar: 0 g

6. Eggs:
Calories: 68 per large egg (cooked)
Sugar: 0.6 g

7. Greek Yogurt (Plain, Non-fat):
Calories: 59 per 100g
Sugar: 4 g

8. Cottage Cheese (Low-fat):
Calories: 206 per cup
Sugar: 6 g

9. Lean Ground Beef (90% Lean):
Calories: 184 per 3.5 oz (cooked)
Sugar: 0 g

10. Lentils:
Calories: 116 per 3.5 oz (cooked)
Sugar: 2 g

11. Pork Loin (Trimmed):
Calories: 143 per 3.5 oz (cooked)
Sugar: 0 g

12. Quinoa:
Calories: 120 per 1 cup (cooked)
Sugar: 0.9 g

13. Skinless Turkey Sausage:
Calories: 150 per 3.5 oz (cooked)
Sugar: 0 g

14. Cod:
Calories: 105 per 3.5 oz (cooked)
Sugar: 0 g

15. Lean Ham:
Calories: 143 per 3.5 oz (cooked)
Sugar: 0 g

16. Edamame:
Calories: 122 per cup (cooked)
Sugar: 2 g

17. Skinless, Boneless Chicken Thighs:
Calories: 165 per 3.5 oz (cooked)
Sugar: 0 g

18. Bison:
Calories: 143 per 3.5 oz (cooked)
Sugar: 0 g

19. Mackerel:
Calories: 305 per 3.5 oz (cooked)
Sugar: 0 g

20. Chicken Drumsticks (Skinless):
Calories: 165 per 3.5 oz (cooked)
Sugar: 0 g

Fats and Oil

1. Olive Oil:
Calories: 119 per tablespoon
Sugar: 0 g

2. Avocado:
Calories: 322 per avocado
Sugar: 1.7 g

3. Almonds:
Calories: 7 per almond
Sugar: 0.2 g

4. Chia Seeds:
Calories: 138 per ounce
Sugar: 0 g

5. Flaxseeds:
Calories: 55 per tablespoon
Sugar: 0.2 g

6. Walnuts:
Calories: 185 per ounce
Sugar: 0.7 g

7. Peanut Butter (Natural, Unsweetened):
Calories: 94 per tablespoon
Sugar: 1.7 g

8. Coconut Oil:
Calories: 117 per tablespoon
Sugar: 0 g

9. Salmon (Wild-Caught):
Calories: 206 per 3.5 oz (cooked)
Sugar: 0 g

10. Dark Chocolate (70-85% Cocoa):
Calories: 160 per ounce
Sugar: 6.7 g

11. Hemp Seeds:
Calories: 166 per ounce
Sugar: 0.2 g

12. Pistachios:
Calories: 156 per ounce
Sugar: 2.2 g

13. Sunflower Seeds:
Calories: 204 per ounce
Sugar: 0.7 g

14. Greek Yogurt (Full-Fat, Plain):
Calories: 69 per 100g
Sugar: 4.1 g

15. Sesame Oil:
Calories: 120 per tablespoon
Sugar: 0 g

16. Pecans:
Calories: 193 per ounce
Sugar: 1.1 g

17. Cashews:
Calories: 155 per ounce
Sugar: 1.7 g

18. Sardines (in Olive Oil):
Calories: 191 per 3.5 oz
Sugar: 0 g

19. Pumpkin Seeds:
Calories: 151 per ounce
Sugar: 0.9 g

20. Butter (Grass-Fed, Unsalted):
Calories: 102 per tablespoon
Sugar: 0 g

Legumes and Grains

1. Lentils:
Calories: 230 per cup (cooked)
Sugar: 1 g
Protein: 18 g

2. Chickpeas:
Calories: 269 per cup (cooked)
Sugar: 4 g
Protein: 14.5 g

3. Black Beans:
Calories: 227 per cup (cooked)
Sugar: 0 g
Protein: 15.2 g

4. Quinoa:
Calories: 222 per cup (cooked)
Sugar: 0.9 g
Protein: 8 g

5. Brown Rice:
Calories: 215 per cup (cooked)
Sugar: 0.7 g
Protein: 5 g

6. Barley:
Calories: 193 per cup (cooked)
Sugar: 0.8 g
Protein: 3.5 g

7. Oats (Steel-Cut):
Calories: 150 per cup (cooked)
Sugar: 0.4 g
Protein: 5 g

8. Bulgur:
Calories: 151 per cup (cooked)
Sugar: 0.1 g
Protein: 6 g

9. Farro:
Calories: 337 per cup (cooked)
Sugar: 0.4 g
Protein: 14 g

10. Whole Wheat Pasta:
- Calories: 174 per cup (cooked)
- Sugar: 0.8 g
- Protein: 7.5 g

11. Black Rice (Forbidden Rice):
- Calories: 215 per cup (cooked)
- Sugar: 0.6 g
- Protein: 5 g

12. Buckwheat:
- Calories: 155 per cup (cooked)
- Sugar: 0.2 g
- Protein: 6 g

13. Millet:
- Calories: 207 per cup (cooked)
- Sugar: 0.2 g
- Protein: 6 g

14. Chickpea Flour (Besan):
- Calories: 356 per cup
- Sugar: 4 g
- Protein: 21 g

15. Whole Wheat Bread:
- Calories: 69 per slice
- Sugar: 1 g

- Protein: 3 g

16. Red Lentils:
- Calories: 230 per cup (cooked)
- Sugar: 4 g
- Protein: 16 g

17. Split Peas:
- Calories: 231 per cup (cooked)
- Sugar: 8 g
- Protein: 16 g

18. Wild Rice:
- Calories: 166 per cup (cooked)
- Sugar: 0.3 g
- Protein: 6.5 g

19. Couscous (Whole Wheat):
- Calories: 176 per cup (cooked)
- Sugar: 0.1 g
- Protein: 6 g

20. Amaranth:
- Calories: 251 per cup (cooked)
- Sugar: 1 g
- Protein: 9 g

1. Almond Milk (Unsweetened):
Calories: 13 per cup
Sugar: 0 g

2. Soy Milk (Unsweetened):
Calories: 80 per cup
Sugar: 0 g

3. Coconut Milk (Unsweetened):
Calories: 45 per cup
Sugar: 0 g

4. Cashew Milk (Unsweetened):
Calories: 25 per cup
Sugar: 0 g

5. Oat Milk (Unsweetened):
Calories: 80 per cup
Sugar: 0 g

6. Hemp Milk (Unsweetened):
Calories: 70 per cup
Sugar: 0 g

7. Rice Milk (Unsweetened):
Calories: 120 per cup
Sugar: 0 g

8. Greek Yogurt (Non-Dairy, Unsweetened):
Calories: 59 per 100g
Sugar: 4.1 g

9. Coconut Yogurt (Unsweetened):
Calories: 35 per 100g
Sugar: 1.7 g

10. Almond Yogurt (Unsweetened):
- Calories: 13 per 100g
- Sugar: 0.2 g

11. Soy Yogurt (Unsweetened):
- Calories: 33 per 100g
- Sugar: 1.7 g

12. Flax Milk (Unsweetened):
- Calories: 25 per cup
- Sugar: 0 g

13. Hazelnut Milk (Unsweetened):
- Calories: 50 per cup
- Sugar: 0 g

14. Macadamia Milk (Unsweetened):
- Calories: 50 per cup
- Sugar: 0 g

15. Quinoa Milk (Unsweetened):
- Calories: 70 per cup
- Sugar: 0 g

16. Pea Milk (Unsweetened):
- Calories: 70 per cup
- Sugar: 0 g

17. Cashew Yogurt (Unsweetened):
- Calories: 58 per 100g
- Sugar: 0.1 g

18. Walnut Milk (Unsweetened):
- Calories: 45 per cup
- Sugar: 0 g

19. Sunflower Milk (Unsweetcned):
- Calories: 50 per cup
- Sugar: 0 g

20. Pistachio Milk (Unsweetened):
- Calories: 80 per cup
- Sugar: 0 g

Remember to check labels for added sugars, and choose unsweetened options whenever possible.

Snacks

1. Mixed Nuts (Unsalted):
Calories: 160 per ounce
Sugar: 1 g

2. Fresh Fruit (e.g., Berries, Apple Slices):
Calories: Varies based on the fruit
Sugar: Natural sugars present in the fruit

3. Greek Yogurt (Plain, Non-fat):
Calories: 59 per 100g
Sugar: 4.1 g

4. Cheese Sticks:
Calories: 80 per stick
Sugar: 0 g

5. Hummus with Veggie Sticks (Carrots, Cucumber):
Calories: 70 per 2 tablespoons (hummus)
Sugar: 0 g

6. Hard-Boiled Eggs:
Calories: 68 per large egg
Sugar: 0.6 g

7. Popcorn (Air-Popped):
Calories: 31 per cup
Sugar: 0 g

8. Celery Sticks with Peanut Butter (Unsweetened):
Calories: 98 per 2 tablespoons (peanut butter)
Sugar: 1.7 g

9. Avocado Slices with a Sprinkle of Sea Salt:
Calories: 234 per cup (sliced avocado)
Sugar: 0.7 g

10. Cottage Cheese (Low-fat):
- Calories: 206 per cup
- Sugar: 6 g

11. Seaweed Snacks:
- Calories: 20 per pack
- Sugar: 0 g

12. Cherry Tomatoes with Mozzarella Balls:
- Calories: 27 per 100g (mozzarella balls)
- Sugar: 1 g

13. Almond Butter on Whole Grain Crackers:
- Calories: 98 per 2 tablespoons (almond butter)
- Sugar: 1 g

14. Sugar-Free Jello Cups:
- Calories: 5 per cup
- Sugar: 0 g

15. Veggie Chips (Baked, Not Fried):
- Calories: Varies based on the vegetable
- Sugar: Varies based on the vegetable

16. Edamame (Steamed):
- Calories: 122 per cup
- Sugar: 2 g

17. Dark Chocolate (70-85% Cocoa):
- Calories: 160 per ounce
- Sugar: 6.7 g

18. Rice Cake with Cottage Cheese and Cherry Tomatoes:
- Calories: 70 per rice cake
- Sugar: 1 g

19. Apple Slices with Almond Butter:
- Calories: Varies based on the apple size
- Sugar: Varies based on the apple size

20. Jerky (Turkey or Beef, Low-Sodium):
- Calories: Varies based on the brand
- Sugar: Varies based on the brand

Sweetner and Condiments

1. Stevia (Liquid or Powder):
Calories: 0
Sugar: 0 g

2. Monk Fruit Sweetener:
Calories: 0
Sugar: 0 g

3. Erythritol:
Calories: 0.24 per gram
Sugar: 0 g

4. Xylitol:
Calories: 2.4 per gram
Sugar: 0 g

5. Splenda (Sucralose):
Calories: 3.36 per gram
Sugar: 0 g

6. Agave Nectar (Use Sparingly):
Calories: 60 per tablespoon
Sugar: 16 g

7. Coconut Sugar:
Calories: 45 per tablespoon
Sugar: 5 g

8. Swerve (Erythritol Blend):
Calories: 0
Sugar: 0 g

9. Allulose:
Calories: 0.2 per gram
Sugar: 0 g

10. Maple Syrup (Sugar-Free or Light):
- Calories: 52 per tablespoon
- Sugar: 0 g

11. Mustard:
- Calories: 3 per teaspoon
- Sugar: 0 g

12. Hot Sauce:
- Calories: 0 per teaspoon
- Sugar: 0 g

13. Soy Sauce (Reduced Sodium):
- Calories: 4 per tablespoon
- Sugar: 0.9 g

14. Apple Cider Vinegar:
- Calories: 0 per tablespoon
- Sugar: 0 g

15. Tomato Sauce (No Added Sugar):
- Calories: 20 per 1/2 cup
- Sugar: 4 g

16. Salsa (No Added Sugar):

- Calories: 10 per 2 tablespoons
- Sugar: 2 g

17. Olive Tapenade:
- Calories: 27 per tablespoon
- Sugar: 0 g

18. Pesto Sauce:
- Calories: 58 per tablespoon
- Sugar: 0.2 g

19. Sugar-Free Ketchup:
- Calories: 5 per tablespoon
- Sugar: 0 g

20. Balsamic Vinegar (No Added Sugar):
- Calories: 14 per tablespoon
- Sugar: 2 g

Beverages

1. Water:
Calories: 0
Sugar: 0 g

2. Herbal Tea (Unsweetened):
Calories: 0
Sugar: 0 g

3. Green Tea (Unsweetened):
Calories: 0
Sugar: 0 g

4. Black Coffee (Unsweetened):
Calories: 2 per cup
Sugar: 0 g

5. Sparkling Water (Unsweetened):
Calories: 0
Sugar: 0 g

6. Coconut Water (No Added Sugar):
Calories: 46 per cup
Sugar: 6 g

7. Almond Milk (Unsweetened):
Calories: 13 per cup
Sugar: 0 g

8. Cashew Milk (Unsweetened):
Calories: 25 per cup
Sugar: 0 g

9. Soy Milk (Unsweetened):
Calories: 80 per cup
Sugar: 0 g

10. Buttermilk (Low-Fat):
- Calories: 98 per cup
- Sugar: 12 g

11. Kombucha (No Added Sugar):
- Calories: 30 per cup
- Sugar: 4 g

12. Vegetable Juice (Low-Sodium):

- Calories: 41 per cup
- Sugar: 7 g

13. Tomato Juice (Low-Sodium):
- Calories: 41 per cup
- Sugar: 10 g

14. Iced Green Tea (Unsweetened):
- Calories: 0
- Sugar: 0 g

15. Diet Soda (Sugar-Free):
- Calories: 0
- Sugar: 0 g

16. Sparkling Lemon Water (Unsweetened):
- Calories: 0
- Sugar: 0 g

17. Cranberry Juice (No Added Sugar):
- Calories: 46 per cup
- Sugar: 9 g

18. Lemonade (Sugar-Free):
- Calories: 5 per cup
- Sugar: 0 g

19. Unsweetened Almond Iced Coffee:
- Calories: 15 per cup
- Sugar: 0 g

20. Ginger Tea (Unsweetened):
- Calories: 0
- Sugar: 0 g

Low GI Fruits

Cherries:
GI: 22
Calories (per cup): 87
GL: 6
Sugar (per cup): 18.9 g

Grapefruit:
GI: 25
Calories (per medium grapefruit): 52
GL: 6
Sugar (per medium grapefruit): 8 g

Apricots:
GI: 34
Calories (per apricot): 17
GL: 3
Sugar (per apricot): 3.9 g

Plums:
GI: 39
Calories (per plum): 30
GL: 5
Sugar (per plum): 6.3 g

Peaches:
GI: 42
Calories (per medium peach): 58
GL: 6
Sugar (per medium peach): 13.3 g

Apples:
GI: 36
Calories (per medium apple): 95
GL: 6
Sugar (per medium apple): 19 g

Pears:
GI: 38
Calories (per medium pear): 101
GL: 6
Sugar (per medium pear): 17 g

Oranges:
GI: 42
Calories (per medium orange): 62
GL: 5
Sugar (per medium orange): 12.2 g

Strawberries:
GI: 40
Calories (per cup): 50
GL: 3
Sugar (per cup): 7.4 g

Grapes:
GI: 46
Calories (per cup): 104
GL: 11
Sugar (per cup): 23.4 g

Low GI Vegetables

Broccoli:
GI: 15
Calories (per cup, chopped): 55
GL: 2
Sugar (per cup): 1.5 g

Cauliflower:
GI: 15
Calories (per cup, chopped): 27
GL: 1
Sugar (per cup): 2.4 g

Spinach:
GI: 6
Calories (per cup): 7
GL: 0
Sugar (per cup): 0.9 g

Tomatoes:
GI: 15
Calories (per medium tomato): 22
GL: 2
Sugar (per medium tomato): 4.8 g

Zucchini:
GI: 15
Calories (per cup, sliced): 19
GL: 1
Sugar (per cup): 1.5 g

Peppers (Bell Peppers):
GI: 10
Calories (per medium pepper): 25
GL: 1
Sugar (per medium pepper): 4.2 g

Cabbage:
GI: 10
Calories (per cup, shredded): 22
GL: 1
Sugar (per cup): 2.3 g

Lettuce:
GI: 10
Calories (per cup, shredded): 5
GL: 0
Sugar (per cup): 0.5 g

Asparagus:
GI: 15
Calories (per cup): 27
GL: 2
Sugar (per cup): 2.5 g

Green Beans:
GI: 15
Calories (per cup): 31
GL: 2
Sugar (per cup): 3.6 g

Low GI Legumes and Pulses

Lentils:
GI: 32
Calories (per cup, cooked): 230
GL: 12
Sugar (per cup): 1 g

Chickpeas:
GI: 28
Calories (per cup, cooked): 269
GL: 14
Sugar (per cup): 4 g

Kidney Beans:
GI: 28
Calories (per cup, cooked): 225
GL: 7
Sugar (per cup): 0.3 g

Black Beans:
GI: 30
Calories (per cup, cooked): 227
GL: 7
Sugar (per cup): 0.3 g

Pinto Beans:
GI: 39
Calories (per cup, cooked): 245
GL: 14
Sugar (per cup): 0.3 g

Chickpea Flour (Besan):
GI: 33
Calories (per cup): 356
GL: 19
Sugar (per cup): 4 g

Red Lentils:
GI: 26
Calories (per cup, cooked): 230
GL: 12
Sugar (per cup): 4 g

Split Peas:
GI: 25
Calories (per cup, cooked): 231
GL: 12
Sugar (per cup): 8 g

Soybeans (Edamame):
GI: 15
Calories (per cup, cooked): 298
GL: 6
Sugar (per cup): 6 g

Black-eyed Peas:
GI: 33
Calories (per cup, cooked): 220
GL: 17
Sugar (per cup): 5 g

Low GI whole grains

Quinoa:
GI: 53
Calories (per cup, cooked): 222
GL: 13
Sugar (per cup): 1.6 g

Barley:
GI: 28
Calories (per cup, cooked): 193
GL: 7
Sugar (per cup): 0.8 g

Bulgur:
GI: 48
Calories (per cup, cooked): 151
GL: 12
Sugar (per cup): 0.1 g

Oats (Steel-Cut):
GI: 42
Calories (per cup, cooked): 150
GL: 14
Sugar (per cup): 0.4 g

Brown Rice:
GI: 50
Calories (per cup, cooked): 215
GL: 16
Sugar (per cup): 0.7 g

Farro:
GI: 40
Calories (per cup, cooked): 337
GL: 21
Sugar (per cup): 0.4 g

Whole Wheat Pasta:
GI: 37
Calories (per cup, cooked): 174
GL: 16
Sugar (per cup): 0.8 g

Black Rice (Forbidden Rice):
GI: 42
Calories (per cup, cooked): 215
GL: 18
Sugar (per cup): 0.6 g

Buckwheat:
GI: 49
Calories (per cup, cooked): 155
GL: 13
Sugar (per cup): 0.2 g

Millet:
GI: 71
Calories (per cup, cooked): 207
GL: 23
Sugar (per cup): 0.2 g

Low GI Dairy and Dairy Alternatives

Greek Yogurt (Plain, Non-fat):
GI: 11
Calories (per 100g): 59
GL: 3
Sugar (per 100g): 4.1 g

Milk (Low-Fat):
GI: 32
Calories (per cup): 102
GL: 5
Sugar (per cup): 12 g

Almond Milk (Unsweetened):
GI: 30
Calories (per cup): 13
GL: 1
Sugar (per cup): 0 g

Soy Milk (Unsweetened):
GI: 44
Calories (per cup): 80
GL: 4
Sugar (per cup): 0 g

Coconut Milk (Unsweetened):
GI: 41
Calories (per cup): 45
GL: 5
Sugar (per cup): 0 g

Cashew Milk (Unsweetened):
GI: 25
Calories (per cup): 25
GL: 1
Sugar (per cup): 0 g

Oat Milk (Unsweetened):
GI: 40
Calories (per cup): 80
GL: 4
Sugar (per cup): 0 g

Coconut Yogurt (Unsweetened):
GI: 24
Calories (per 100g): 35
GL: 2
Sugar (per 100g): 1.7 g

Almond Yogurt (Unsweetened):
GI: 25
Calories (per 100g): 13
GL: 1
Sugar (per 100g): 0.2 g

Soy Yogurt (Unsweetened):
GI: 34
Calories (per 100g): 33
GL: 4
Sugar (per 100g): 1.7 g

Low GI Nuts and Seed

Almonds:
GI: 0 (Nuts generally have minimal impact on blood sugar)
Calories (per 1 oz): 160
GL: 0
Sugar (per 1 oz): 1 g

Walnuts:
GI: 0
Calories (per 1 oz): 185
GL: 0
Sugar (per 1 oz): 1 g

Peanuts:
GI: 23
Calories (per 1 oz): 161
GL: 4
Sugar (per 1 oz): 1 g

Cashews:
GI: 22
Calories (per 1 oz): 157
GL: 4
Sugar (per 1 oz): 1 g

Chia Seeds:
GI: 5
Calories (per 1 oz): 138
GL: 1
Sugar (per 1 oz): 0 g

Flaxseeds:
GI: 32
Calories (per 2 tbsp): 74
GL: 2
Sugar (per 2 tbsp): 0.2 g

Sunflower Seeds:
GI: 20
Calories (per 1 oz): 163
GL: 3
Sugar (per 1 oz): 0.3 g

Pumpkin Seeds (Pepitas):
GI: 25
Calories (per 1 oz): 151
GL: 4
Sugar (per 1 oz): 0.3 g

Hazelnuts:
GI: 0
Calories (per 1 oz): 176
GL: 0
Sugar (per 1 oz): 1 g

Pistachios:
GI: 0
Calories (per 1 oz): 159
GL: 0
Sugar (per 1 oz): 2 g

Low GI proteins

Chicken Breast (Grilled):
GI: 0
Calories (per 3 oz): 165
GL: 0
Sugar (per 3 oz): 0 g

Turkey (Roasted):
GI: 0
Calories (per 3 oz): 135
GL: 0
Sugar (per 3 oz): 0 g

Fish (Salmon, Baked):
GI: 0
Calories (per 3 oz): 155
GL: 0
Sugar (per 3 oz): 0 g

Tofu:
GI: 15
Calories (per 3 oz): 70
GL: 1
Sugar (per 3 oz): 0 g

Eggs (Hard-Boiled):
GI: 0
Calories (per large egg): 68
GL: 0
Sugar (per large egg): 0.6 g

Lentils (Cooked):
GI: 32
Calories (per cup): 230
GL: 12
Sugar (per cup): 1 g

Chickpeas (Cooked):
GI: 28
Calories (per cup): 269
GL: 14
Sugar (per cup): 4 g

Black Beans (Cooked):
GI: 30
Calories (per cup): 227
GL: 7
Sugar (per cup): 0.3 g

Quinoa:
GI: 53
Calories (per cup, cooked): 222
GL: 13
Sugar (per cup): 1.6 g

Greek Yogurt (Plain, Non-fat):
GI: 11
Calories (per 100g): 59
GL: 3
Sugar (per 100g): 4.1 g

Low GI fats and Oil

Olive Oil:
Calories (per tablespoon): 119
Type of Fat: Monounsaturated
Nutritional Benefits: Rich in heart-healthy monounsaturated fats.

Avocado Oil:
Calories (per tablespoon): 124
Type of Fat: Monounsaturated
Nutritional Benefits: Contains monounsaturated fats and various antioxidants.

Coconut Oil:
Calories (per tablespoon): 121
Type of Fat: Saturated
Nutritional Benefits: Contains medium-chain triglycerides (MCTs) and has various uses.

Flaxseed Oil:
Calories (per tablespoon): 120
Type of Fat: Polyunsaturated (Omega-3)
Nutritional Benefits: Rich in omega-3 fatty acids.

Walnut Oil:
Calories (per tablespoon): 120
Type of Fat: Polyunsaturated (Omega-3)
Nutritional Benefits: Contains omega-3 fatty acids.

Sesame Oil:
Calories (per tablespoon): 120
Type of Fat: Monounsaturated and Polyunsaturated
Nutritional Benefits: Adds a rich flavor to dishes.

Canola Oil:
Calories (per tablespoon): 124
Type of Fat: Monounsaturated and Polyunsaturated
Nutritional Benefits: Low in saturated fat and a good source of omega-3 fatty acids.

Ghee (Clarified Butter):
Calories (per tablespoon): 112
Type of Fat: Saturated
Nutritional Benefits: Lactose-free and has a high smoke point.

Sunflower Oil:
Calories (per tablespoon): 124
Type of Fat: Monounsaturated and Polyunsaturated
Nutritional Benefits: Contains vitamin E and low in saturated fat.

Peanut Oil:
Calories (per tablespoon): 119
Type of Fat: Monounsaturated and Polyunsaturated
Nutritional Benefits: Has a high smoke point and is commonly used in frying.

Hummus with Vegetable Sticks:
GI: 6
Calories (per serving): 100
GL: 1
Sugar (per serving): 0 g

Greek Yogurt with Berries:
GI: 11
Calories (per serving): 150
GL: 3
Sugar (per serving): 10 g

Nuts (Almonds, Walnuts, or Pistachios):
GI: 0
Calories (per 1 oz serving): Varies (e.g., Almonds - 160 calories)
GL: 0
Sugar (per 1 oz serving): Varies (e.g., Almonds - 1 g)

Cheese and Whole Grain Crackers:
GI: 22
Calories (per serving): 150
GL: 4
Sugar (per serving): 0 g

Hard-Boiled Eggs:
GI: 0
Calories (per egg): 68
GL: 0
Sugar (per egg): 0.6 g

Vegetable Chips (Baked):
GI: Varies based on vegetables
Calories (per serving): Varies
GL: Varies
Sugar (per serving): Varies

Edamame (Steamed Soybeans):
GI: 15
Calories (per 1 cup): 189
GL: 4
Sugar (per 1 cup): 3 g

Dark Chocolate (70% cocoa or higher):
GI: 20
Calories (per 1 oz): 170
GL: 3
Sugar (per 1 oz): 6 g

Cottage Cheese with Pineapple:
GI: 22
Calories (per serving): 206
GL: 5
Sugar (per serving): 16 g

Trail Mix with Dried Fruits and Nuts:
GI: Varies based on ingredients
Calories (per 1 oz serving): Varies
GL: Varies
Sugar (per 1 oz serving): Varies

Green Tea:
GI: 0
Calories (per 8 oz): 0
GL: 0
Sugar (per 8 oz): 0 g

Black Coffee (Unsweetened):
GI: 0
Calories (per 8 oz): 2
GL: 0
Sugar (per 8 oz): 0 g

Herbal Tea (Unsweetened):
GI: 0
Calories (per 8 oz): 0
GL: 0
Sugar (per 8 oz): 0 g

Water (Still or Sparkling):
GI: 0
Calories (per 8 oz): 0
GL: 0
Sugar (per 8 oz): 0 g

Almond Milk (Unsweetened):
GI: 30
Calories (per cup): 13
GL: 1
Sugar (per cup): 0 g

Coconut Water (Unsweetened):
GI: 41
Calories (per cup): 46
GL: 5
Sugar (per cup): 6 g

Vegetable Juice (Low-Sodium):
GI: Varies
Calories (per cup): Varies
GL: Varies
Sugar (per cup): Varies

Tomato Juice (Low-Sodium):
GI: 38
Calories (per cup): 41
GL: 7
Sugar (per cup): 9 g

Iced Green Tea (Unsweetened):
GI: 0
Calories (per 8 oz): 0
GL: 0
Sugar (per 8 oz): 0 g

Kombucha (Unsweetened):
GI: Varies
Calories (per cup): Varies
GL: Varies
Sugar (per cup): Varies

Low GI Seafood

Salmon (Grilled):
GI: 0
Calories (per 3 oz): 180
GL: 0
Sugar (per 3 oz): 0 g

Shrimp (Steamed):
GI: 0
Calories (per 3 oz): 84
GL: 0
Sugar (per 3 oz): 0 g

Tuna (Fresh, Raw):
GI: 0
Calories (per 3 oz): 93
GL: 0
Sugar (per 3 oz): 0 g

Cod (Baked):
GI: 0
Calories (per 3 oz): 89
GL: 0
Sugar (per 3 oz): 0 g

Sardines (Canned in Water):
GI: 0
Calories (per 3 oz): 177
GL: 0
Sugar (per 3 oz): 0 g

Crab (Steamed):
GI: 0
Calories (per 3 oz): 98
GL: 0
Sugar (per 3 oz): 0 g

Lobster (Boiled):
GI: 0
Calories (per 3 oz): 82
GL: 0
Sugar (per 3 oz): 0 g

Mackerel (Grilled):
GI: 0
Calories (per 3 oz): 230
GL: 0
Sugar (per 3 oz): 0 g

Clams (Steamed):
GI: 0
Calories (per 3 oz): 126
GL: 0
Sugar (per 3 oz): 0 g

Halibut (Baked):
GI: 0
Calories (per 3 oz): 93
GL: 0
Sugar (per 3 oz): 0 g

Low GI Soup and Broths

Chicken Broth (Homemade):
GI: 0
Calories (per cup): 12
GL: 0
Sugar (per cup): 0 g

Vegetable Soup (No Added Starches):
GI: Varies
Calories (per cup): Varies
GL: Varies
Sugar (per cup): Varies

Tomato Soup (No Added Sugar):
GI: 38
Calories (per cup): 74
GL: 7
Sugar (per cup): 5 g

Miso Soup:
GI: Varies
Calories (per cup): Varies
GL: Varies
Sugar (per cup): Varies

Clear Fish Broth:
GI: 0
Calories (per cup): 16
GL: 0
Sugar (per cup): 0 g

Lentil Soup (Without Added High-GI Ingredients):
GI: 29
Calories (per cup): 200
GL: 12
Sugar (per cup): 3 g

Minestrone Soup (No Pasta or High-GI Ingredients):
GI: Varies
Calories (per cup): Varies
GL: Varies
Sugar (per cup): Varies

Gazpacho (Tomato-based Cold Soup):
GI: Varies
Calories (per cup): Varies
GL: Varies
Sugar (per cup): Varies

Bone Broth (Homemade):
GI: 0
Calories (per cup): 86
GL: 0
Sugar (per cup): 0 g

Spinach and Kale Soup:
GI: Varies
Calories (per cup): Varies
GL: Varies
Sugar (per cup): Varies

Cinnamon:
GI: 0
Calories (per teaspoon): 6
GL: 0
Sugar (per teaspoon): 0 g

Turmeric:
GI: 0
Calories (per teaspoon): 9
GL: 0
Sugar (per teaspoon): 0 g

Basil:
GI: 0
Calories (per tablespoon, fresh): 1
GL: 0
Sugar (per tablespoon, fresh): 0 g

Oregano:
GI: 0
Calories (per teaspoon, dried): 5
GL: 0
Sugar (per teaspoon, dried): 0 g

Garlic Powder:
GI: 0
Calories (per teaspoon): 10
GL: 0
Sugar (per teaspoon): 0 g

Ginger:
GI: 0
Calories (per teaspoon, fresh): 2
GL: 0
Sugar (per teaspoon, fresh): 0 g

Parsley:
GI: 0
Calories (per tablespoon, fresh): 1
GL: 0
Sugar (per tablespoon, fresh): 0 g

Rosemary:
GI: 0
Calories (per teaspoon, dried): 2
GL: 0
Sugar (per teaspoon, dried): 0 g

Cayenne Pepper:
GI: 0
Calories (per teaspoon): 6
GL: 0
Sugar (per teaspoon): 0 g

Thyme:
GI: 0
Calories (per teaspoon, dried): 3
GL: 0
Sugar (per teaspoon, dried): 0 g

Low GI Sweeteners

Stevia:
GI: 0
Calories (per teaspoon): 0
GL: 0
Sugar (per teaspoon): 0 g

Monk Fruit Sweetener:
GI: 0
Calories (per teaspoon): 0
GL: 0
Sugar (per teaspoon): 0 g

Erythritol:
GI: 1
Calories (per teaspoon): 0.2
GL: 0
Sugar (per teaspoon): 0 g

Xylitol:
GI: 7
Calories (per teaspoon): 9.6
GL: 1
Sugar (per teaspoon): 0 g

Agave Nectar (in moderation):
GI: 15
Calories (per teaspoon): 20
GL: 3
Sugar (per teaspoon): 5 g

Coconut Sugar:
GI: 54
Calories (per teaspoon): 15
GL: 8
Sugar (per teaspoon): 4 g

Allulose:
GI: 0
Calories (per teaspoon): 0.2
GL: 0
Sugar (per teaspoon): 0 g

Tagatose:
GI: 3
Calories (per teaspoon): 1.2
GL: 0
Sugar (per teaspoon): 0 g

Yacon Syrup:
GI: 1
Calories (per teaspoon): 7
GL: 0
Sugar (per teaspoon): 1.7 g

Inulin (Chicory Root Fiber):
GI: 0
Calories (per teaspoon): 3
GL: 0
Sugar (per teaspoon): 0 g

Low GI Condiments and Sauces

Mustard:
GI: 0
Calories (per tablespoon): 3
GL: 0
Sugar (per tablespoon): 0 g

Soy Sauce (Reduced Sodium):
GI: 0
Calories (per tablespoon): 10
GL: 0
Sugar (per tablespoon): 1 g

Vinegar (White or Apple Cider):
GI: 0
Calories (per tablespoon): 3
GL: 0
Sugar (per tablespoon): 0 g

Hot Sauce (e.g., Tabasco):
GI: 0
Calories (per tablespoon): 0
GL: 0
Sugar (per tablespoon): 0 g

Pesto (Basil, Olive Oil, Garlic):
GI: Varies
Calories (per tablespoon): Varies
GL: Varies
Sugar (per tablespoon): Varies

Tahini (Pure Sesame Paste):
GI: 0
Calories (per tablespoon): 89
GL: 0
Sugar (per tablespoon): 0 g

Guacamole (Homemade):
GI: Varies
Calories (per tablespoon): Varies
GL: Varies
Sugar (per tablespoon): Varies

Salsa (Fresh, Tomato-based):
GI: Varies
Calories (per tablespoon): Varies
GL: Varies
Sugar (per tablespoon): Varies

Hummus (Chickpea-based):
GI: 6
Calories (per tablespoon): 27
GL: 2
Sugar (per tablespoon): 0 g

Worcestershire Sauce:
GI: 0
Calories (per tablespoon): 12
GL: 0
Sugar (per tablespoon): 1 g

Low GI Spreads and Dips

Avocado Spread (Mashed):
GI: 0
Calories (per tablespoon): 20
GL: 0
Sugar (per tablespoon): 0.2 g

Olive Tapenade:
GI: 0
Calories (per tablespoon): 30
GL: 0
Sugar (per tablespoon): 0 g

Greek Yogurt Dip (Plain, Non-fat):
GI: 11
Calories (per tablespoon): 7
GL: 1
Sugar (per tablespoon): 0.6 g

Hummus (Chickpea-based):
GI: 6
Calories (per tablespoon): 27
GL: 2
Sugar (per tablespoon): 0 g

Guacamole (Homemade):
GI: Varies
Calories (per tablespoon): Varies
GL: Varies
Sugar (per tablespoon): Varies

Tzatziki (Greek Yogurt and Cucumber Dip):
GI: Varies
Calories (per tablespoon): Varies
GL: Varies
Sugar (per tablespoon): Varies

Nut Butter (Almond, Peanut, or Cashew):
GI: 0
Calories (per tablespoon): Varies
GL: Varies
Sugar (per tablespoon): Varies

Salsa (Fresh, Tomato-based):
GI: Varies
Calories (per tablespoon): Varies
GL: Varies
Sugar (per tablespoon): Varies

Baba Ganoush (Roasted Eggplant Dip):
GI: Varies
Calories (per tablespoon): Varies
GL: Varies
Sugar (per tablespoon): Varies

Ricotta Cheese (Low-fat):
GI: 27
Calories (per tablespoon): 14
GL: 4
Sugar (per tablespoon): 0.2 g

Balsamic Vinaigrette Dressing (Homemade):
GI: 6
Calories (per tablespoon): 43
GL: 3
Sugar (per tablespoon): 3 g

Olive Oil and Lemon Marinade:
GI: 0
Calories (per tablespoon): 120
GL: 0
Sugar (per tablespoon): 0 g

Greek Yogurt Caesar Dressing:
GI: 11
Calories (per tablespoon): 19
GL: 1
Sugar (per tablespoon): 1 g

Tahini and Lemon Dressing:
GI: 0
Calories (per tablespoon): 89
GL: 0
Sugar (per tablespoon): 0 g

Asian Ginger Sesame Marinade:
GI: Varies
Calories (per tablespoon): Varies
GL: Varies
Sugar (per tablespoon): Varies

Yogurt and Dill Marinade:
GI: Varies
Calories (per tablespoon): Varies
GL: Varies
Sugar (per tablespoon): Varies

Avocado Lime Dressing:
GI: 0
Calories (per tablespoon): 32
GL: 0
Sugar (per tablespoon): 0.3 g

Soy Ginger Dressing (Low-sodium):
GI: 0
Calories (per tablespoon): 23
GL: 0
Sugar (per tablespoon): 1 g

Mustard Dijon Dressing:
GI: 0
Calories (per tablespoon): 53
GL: 0
Sugar (per tablespoon): 0.3 g

Cilantro Lime Marinade:
GI: Varies
Calories (per tablespoon): Varies
GL: Varies
Sugar (per tablespoon): Varies

Low GI Baking and Cooking Ingredients

Almond Flour:
GI: 0
Calories (per 1/4 cup): 180
GL: 0
Sugar (per 1/4 cup): 0 g

Coconut Flour:
GI: 0
Calories (per 1/4 cup): 120
GL: 0
Sugar (per 1/4 cup): 4 g

Stevia (Natural Sweetener):
GI: 0
Calories (per teaspoon): 0
GL: 0
Sugar (per teaspoon): 0 g

Unsweetened Cocoa Powder:
GI: 0
Calories (per tablespoon): 12
GL: 0
Sugar (per tablespoon): 0 g

Chia Seeds:
GI: 0
Calories (per tablespoon): 69
GL: 0
Sugar (per tablespoon): 0 g

Flaxseed Meal:
GI: 0
Calories (per tablespoon): 37
GL: 0
Sugar (per tablespoon): 0 g

Erythritol (Sugar Substitute):
GI: 1
Calories (per teaspoon): 0
GL: 0
Sugar (per teaspoon): 0 g

Pure Vanilla Extract:
GI: 0
Calories (per teaspoon): 12
GL: 0
Sugar (per teaspoon): 0 g

Cinnamon (Ground):
GI: 0
Calories (per teaspoon): 6
GL: 0
Sugar (per teaspoon): 0 g

Psyllium Husk Powder:
GI: 0
Calories (per teaspoon): 10
GL: 0
Sugar (per teaspoon): 0 g

Breakfast

1. Greek Yogurt Parfait:

Ingredients:

1 cup Greek yogurt (unsweetened)

1/2 cup mixed berries (blueberries, strawberries, raspberries)

1 tablespoon chia seeds

1 tablespoon chopped nuts (almonds or walnuts)

1 teaspoon honey or stevia (optional)

Preparation:

1. In a glass or bowl, layer Greek yogurt at the bottom.
2. Add a layer of mixed berries.
3. Sprinkle chia seeds and chopped nuts on top.
4. Drizzle with honey or add stevia for sweetness (optional).
5. Repeat layers if desired.

Prep Time: 5 minutes

Nutritional Information:

GI: Varies

Calories: Approximately 250

GL: Varies

Sugar: Varies

2. Vegetable Omelette with Avocado:
Ingredients:
2 large eggs
1/4 cup diced bell peppers (mixed colors)
1/4 cup diced tomatoes
1/4 cup spinach, chopped
1/4 cup feta cheese (optional)
1/2 avocado, sliced

Preparation:
1. Whisk eggs in a bowl and season with salt and pepper.
2. Heat a non-stick pan over medium heat.
3. Pour eggs into the pan and add vegetables.
4. Cook until the edges set, then fold the omelette.
5. Top with feta cheese and serve with sliced avocado.

Prep Time: 10 minutes

Nutritional Information:
GI: 0
Calories: Approximately 350
GL: 0
Sugar: 2 g

3. Chia Seed Pudding:
Ingredients:
2 tablespoons chia seeds
1 cup almond milk (unsweetened)
1/2 teaspoon vanilla extract
1 tablespoon sliced almonds

Fresh berries for topping

Preparation:

1. In a bowl, mix chia seeds, almond milk, and vanilla extract.
2. Stir well and refrigerate overnight or for at least 4 hours.
3. Before serving, top with sliced almonds and fresh berries.

Prep Time: 5 minutes (+ refrigeration time)

Nutritional Information:

GI: 0
Calories: Approximately 200
GL: 0
Sugar: 1 g

4. Quinoa Breakfast Bowl:

Ingredients:
1/2 cup cooked quinoa
1/4 cup Greek yogurt (unsweetened)
1/2 banana, sliced
1 tablespoon almond butter
1 tablespoon hemp seeds

Preparation:

1. In a bowl, layer cooked quinoa.
2. Add a dollop of Greek yogurt.
3. Top with banana slices, almond butter, and hemp seeds.

Prep Time: 15 minutes (if quinoa is pre-cooked)

Nutritional Information:
GI: Varies
Calories: Approximately 350
GL: Varies
Sugar: Varies

5. Sweet Potato Toast with Avocado:

Ingredients:
1 large sweet potato, sliced into rounds
1/2 avocado, mashed
Cherry tomatoes, sliced
Sprinkle of black sesame seeds
Salt and pepper to taste

Preparation:
1. Toast sweet potato rounds until tender.
2. Spread mashed avocado on each round.
3. Top with sliced cherry tomatoes and sprinkle with sesame seeds.
4. Season with salt and pepper to taste.

Prep Time: 20 minutes

Nutritional Information:
GI: Varies
Calories: Approximately 300
GL: Varies
Sugar: Varies

1. Quinoa Salad with Chickpeas and Avocado:
Ingredients:
1 cup cooked quinoa
1/2 cup chickpeas (canned, drained)
1/2 avocado, diced
Cherry tomatoes, halved
Cucumber, diced
Fresh cilantro, chopped
Lemon vinaigrette dressing (olive oil, lemon juice, salt, pepper)

Preparation:
In a bowl, combine cooked quinoa, chickpeas, avocado, tomatoes, cucumber, and cilantro.
Drizzle with lemon vinaigrette dressing and toss until well combined.

Prep Time: 15 minutes

Nutritional Information:
GI: Varies
Calories: Approximately 400
GL: Varies
Sugar: Varies

2. Grilled Chicken and Vegetable Skewers:
Ingredients:
Chicken breast, cut into cubes
Bell peppers (various colors), sliced
Cherry tomatoes
Red onion, sliced
Zucchini, sliced

Olive oil, garlic, herbs for marinade

Preparation:
1. Marinate chicken cubes in olive oil, minced garlic, and herbs.
2. Thread chicken and vegetables onto skewers.
3. Grill until chicken is cooked through and vegetables are tender.

Prep Time: 30 minutes

Nutritional Information:
GI: Varies
Calories: Approximately 350
GL: Varies
Sugar: Varies

3. Salmon and Quinoa Bowl:
Ingredients:
Grilled salmon fillet
1 cup cooked quinoa
Steamed broccoli florets
Sliced avocado
Lemon wedges
Dill and black pepper for seasoning

Preparation:
1. Place cooked quinoa in a bowl.
2. Top with grilled salmon, steamed broccoli, and avocado slices.
3. Season with dill, black pepper, and a squeeze of lemon.

Prep Time: 20 minutes

Nutritional Information:
GI: Varies
Calories: Approximately 400
GL: Varies
Sugar: Varies

4. Vegetarian Stir-Fry with Tofu:
Ingredients:
Firm tofu, cubed
Mixed stir-fry vegetables (bell peppers, broccoli, snap peas)
Low-sodium soy sauce
Ginger and garlic, minced
Sesame oil for cooking

Preparation:
1. Sauté tofu in sesame oil until golden brown.
2. Add minced ginger and garlic, followed by mixed vegetables.
3. Stir in low-sodium soy sauce until vegetables are tender.

Prep Time: 25 minutes

Nutritional Information:
GI: Varies
Calories: Approximately 300
GL: Varies
Sugar: Varies

5. Turkey and Black Bean Lettuce Wraps:
Ingredients:
Ground turkey
Black beans (canned, drained)
Lettuce leaves for wraps
Salsa
Avocado, sliced
Cilantro for garnish

Preparation:
1. Cook ground turkey until browned.
2. Stir in black beans and salsa.
3. Spoon the mixture into lettuce leaves.
4. Top with sliced avocado and garnish with cilantro.

Prep Time: 20 minutes

Nutritional Information:
GI: Varies
Calories: Approximately 350
GL: Varies
Sugar: Varies

1. Grilled Lemon Herb Chicken with Roasted Vegetables:

Ingredients:
Chicken breasts
Zucchini, sliced
Cherry tomatoes
Red onion, sliced
Olive oil, lemon juice, garlic, rosemary, thyme for marinade
Salt and pepper to taste

Preparation:
Marinate chicken in a mixture of olive oil, lemon juice, minced garlic, rosemary, and thyme.
Grill chicken until cooked through.
Roast vegetables with olive oil, salt, and pepper.
Serve chicken over roasted vegetables.

Prep Time: 40 minutes

Nutritional Information:
GI: Varies
Calories: Approximately 400
GL: Varies
Sugar: Varies

2. Spaghetti Squash with Tomato and Basil Sauce:

Ingredients:
Spaghetti squash
Cherry tomatoes, halved
Fresh basil, chopped

Garlic, minced
Olive oil, salt, and pepper

Preparation:
1. Roast spaghetti squash until tender and scrape into strands.
2. Sauté garlic in olive oil, add cherry tomatoes and cook until softened.
3. Toss spaghetti squash with the tomato mixture.
4. Garnish with fresh basil.

Prep Time: 45 minutes

Nutritional Information:
GI: Varies
Calories: Approximately 250
GL: Varies
Sugar: Varies

3. Salmon and Asparagus Foil Packets:
Ingredients:
Salmon fillets
Asparagus spears
Lemon slices
Garlic, minced
Dill, salt, and pepper

Preparation:
1. Place salmon, asparagus, lemon slices, and minced garlic on a foil sheet.
2. Season with dill, salt, and pepper.

3. Seal the foil into packets and bake until salmon is cooked.

Prep Time: 30 minutes

Nutritional Information:
GI: Varies
Calories: Approximately 350
GL: Varies
Sugar: Varies

4. Vegetarian Quinoa Stuffed Peppers:
Ingredients:
Bell peppers, halved
Cooked quinoa
Black beans (canned, drained)
Corn kernels
Salsa
Shredded cheese (optional)

Preparation:
Mix cooked quinoa with black beans, corn, and salsa.
Stuff bell peppers with the quinoa mixture.
Top with shredded cheese (optional) and bake until peppers are tender.

Prep Time: 35 minutes

Nutritional Information:
GI: Varies
Calories: Approximately 300
GL: Varies
Sugar: Varies

5. Eggplant and Chickpea Curry:

Ingredients:
Eggplant, diced
Chickpeas (canned, drained)
Onion, chopped
Tomatoes, diced
Coconut milk
Curry spices (turmeric, cumin, coriander)
Garlic and ginger, minced
Fresh cilantro for garnish

Preparation:
Sauté onion, garlic, and ginger in a pan.
Add eggplant, chickpeas, tomatoes, and curry spices.
Pour in coconut milk and simmer until vegetables are tender.
Garnish with fresh cilantro.

Prep Time: 40 minutes

Nutritional Information:
GI: Varies
Calories: Approximately 350
GL: Varies
Sugar: Varies

Snacks

1. Greek Yogurt with Berries and Almonds:
Ingredients:
1 cup Greek yogurt (unsweetened)
Mixed berries (blueberries, strawberries)
Almonds, sliced
Drizzle of honey or stevia (optional)

Preparation:
Spoon Greek yogurt into a bowl.
Top with mixed berries and sliced almonds.
Drizzle with honey or add stevia for sweetness (optional).

Prep Time: 5 minutes

Nutritional Information:
GI: Varies
Calories: Approximately 200
GL: Varies
Sugar: Varies

2. Veggie Sticks with Hummus:
Ingredients:
Carrot, cucumber, and bell pepper sticks
Hummus (store-bought or homemade)

Preparation:
Cut vegetables into sticks.
Serve with a side of hummus for dipping.

Prep Time: 10 minutes

Nutritional Information:
GI: Varies
Calories: Approximately 150
GL: Varies
Sugar: Varies

3. Chia Seed Pudding with Mango:
Ingredients:
2 tablespoons chia seeds
1 cup almond milk (unsweetened)
1/2 teaspoon vanilla extract
Fresh mango, diced

Preparation:
1. In a jar, mix chia seeds, almond milk, and vanilla extract.
2. Refrigerate overnight or for at least 4 hours.
3. Top with fresh mango before serving.

Prep Time: 5 minutes (+ refrigeration time)

Nutritional Information:
GI: Varies
Calories: Approximately 250
GL: Varies
Sugar: Varies

4. Whole Grain Crackers with Avocado and Tomato:
Ingredients:
Whole grain crackers
Avocado, mashed
Cherry tomatoes, sliced

Sprinkle of black pepper

Preparation:
1. Spread mashed avocado on whole grain crackers.
2. Top with sliced cherry tomatoes.
3. Sprinkle with black pepper.

Prep Time: 10 minutes

Nutritional Information:
GI: Varies
Calories: Approximately 180
GL: Varies
Sugar: Varies

5. Roasted Chickpeas:
Ingredients:
Canned chickpeas, drained and rinsed
Olive oil
Paprika, cumin, garlic powder, salt, and pepper

Preparation:
Toss chickpeas with olive oil and spices.
Roast in the oven until crunchy.

Prep Time: 30 minutes

Nutritional Information:
GI: Varies
Calories: Approximately 150
GL: Varies
Sugar: Varies

1. Chia Seed and Berry Parfait:
Ingredients:
2 tablespoons chia seeds
1 cup almond milk (unsweetened)
Mixed berries (blueberries, raspberries, strawberries)
Unsweetened coconut flakes

Preparation:
Mix chia seeds and almond milk in a jar.
Refrigerate overnight or for at least 4 hours.
Layer chia pudding with mixed berries.
Top with unsweetened coconut flakes.

Prep Time: 5 minutes (+ refrigeration time)

Nutritional Information:
GI: Varies
Calories: Approximately 200
GL: Varies
Sugar: Varies

2. Baked Apples with Cinnamon and Walnuts:
Ingredients:
Apples, cored and sliced
Cinnamon
Chopped walnuts
Greek yogurt (unsweetened, for serving)

Preparation:
1. Preheat the oven to 375°F (190°C).
2. Place apple slices in a baking dish.

3. Sprinkle with cinnamon and chopped walnuts.
4. Bake until apples are tender.
5. Serve with a dollop of Greek yogurt.

Prep Time: 30 minutes

Nutritional Information:
GI: Varies
Calories: Approximately 150
GL: Varies
Sugar: Varies

3. Dark Chocolate-Dipped Strawberries:
Ingredients:
Fresh strawberries
Dark chocolate (70% cocoa or higher)

Preparation:
1. Melt dark chocolate in a heatproof bowl.
2. Dip each strawberry into the melted chocolate.
3. Place on parchment paper and let it cool.

Prep Time: 15 minutes

Nutritional Information:
GI: Varies
Calories: Approximately 100
GL: Varies
Sugar: Varies

4. Coconut and Almond Energy Bites:
Ingredients:
Almond butter
Shredded coconut (unsweetened)
Almond flour
Vanilla extract
Chia seeds

Preparation:
1. Mix almond butter, shredded coconut, almond flour, vanilla extract, and chia seeds in a bowl.
2. Form into bite-sized balls.
3. Chill in the refrigerator before serving.

Prep Time: 20 minutes

Nutritional Information:
GI: Varies
Calories: Approximately 120 per bite
GL: Varies
Sugar: Varies

5. Yogurt and Berry Popsicles:
Ingredients:
Greek yogurt (unsweetened)
Mixed berries (blueberries, strawberries, raspberries)
Honey or stevia (optional)

Preparation:
1. Mix Greek yogurt with berries and sweetener if desired.
2. Pour the mixture into popsicle molds.

3. Freeze until solid.

Prep Time: 10 minutes (+ freezing time)

Nutritional Information:
GI: Varies
Calories: Approximately 80 per popsicle
GL: Varies
Sugar: Varies

Smoothies

1. Berry Green Smoothie:
Ingredients:
1 cup mixed berries (blueberries, strawberries, raspberries)
Handful of spinach leaves
1/2 banana
1 cup unsweetened almond milk
Ice cubes

1. **Preparation:**
2. Combine berries, spinach, banana, and almond milk in a blender.
3. Blend until smooth.
4. Add ice cubes and blend again until desired consistency.

Prep Time: 5 minutes
Nutritional Information:
GI: Varies
Calories: Approximately 150
GL: Varies
Sugar: Varies

2. Avocado and Kale Smoothie:
Ingredients:
1/2 avocado
Handful of kale leaves
1/2 cucumber, peeled and sliced
1/2 apple, cored
1 cup coconut water

Preparation:
1. Combine avocado, kale, cucumber, apple, and coconut water in a blender.
2. Blend until smooth.

Prep Time: 7 minutes

Nutritional Information:
GI: Varies
Calories: Approximately 180
GL: Varies
Sugar: Varies

3. Pineapple and Ginger Smoothie:
Ingredients:
1 cup fresh pineapple chunks
1/2 inch fresh ginger, peeled
1/2 cup Greek yogurt (unsweetened)
1/2 cup coconut water
Ice cubes

Preparation:
1. Blend pineapple, ginger, Greek yogurt, and coconut water until smooth.
2. Add ice cubes and blend again.

Prep Time: 5 minutes
Nutritional Information:
GI: Varies
Calories: Approximately 160
GL: Varies
Sugar: Varies

4. Chocolate Almond Butter Smoothie:

Ingredients:
1 tablespoon almond butter
1 tablespoon unsweetened cocoa powder
1/2 banana
1 cup unsweetened almond milk
Ice cubes

Preparation:
Blend almond butter, cocoa powder, banana, and almond milk until smooth.
Add ice cubes and blend again.

Prep Time: 5 minutes

Nutritional Information:
GI: Varies
Calories: Approximately 200
GL: Varies
Sugar: Varies

5. Mango Coconut Smoothie:

Ingredients:
1 cup fresh mango chunks
1/2 cup coconut milk (unsweetened)
1/2 cup plain yogurt (unsweetened)

1 tablespoon chia seeds
Ice cubes

Preparation:
Blend mango, coconut milk, yogurt, and chia seeds
until smooth.
Add ice cubes and blend again.

Prep Time: 5 minutes

Nutritional Information:
GI: Varies
Calories: Approximately 180
GL: Varies
Sugar: Varies

CONCLUSION

As we conclude this exploration into the Diabetic Type 2 Grocery and Food List, let's reflect on the empowerment that comes from making informed choices and the impact these choices can have on our overall well-being.

Our daily decisions surrounding food are not merely about sustenance; they are powerful tools that can shape the trajectory of our health. Armed with knowledge about the glycemic impact of various foods, we are now equipped to craft a grocery list that not only satisfies our taste buds but also supports our journey towards better blood sugar control and overall health.

The careful curation of this book is a testament to the understanding that no single approach suits everyone. Each of us is unique, with distinct tastes, preferences, and health considerations. The Diabetic Type 2 Grocery and Food List serves as a versatile canvas upon which individuals can paint their own dietary masterpieces, tailored to their specific needs and goals.

Managing Type 2 Diabetes is not about restrictions; it's about embracing a lifestyle that nourishes both body and spirit. This book encourages a shift in perspective—from viewing dietary adjustments as limitations to recognizing them as opportunities for culinary creativity and well-being. The foods listed here are not mere substitutes; they are delicious, nutritious choices that contribute to a vibrant and fulfilling life.

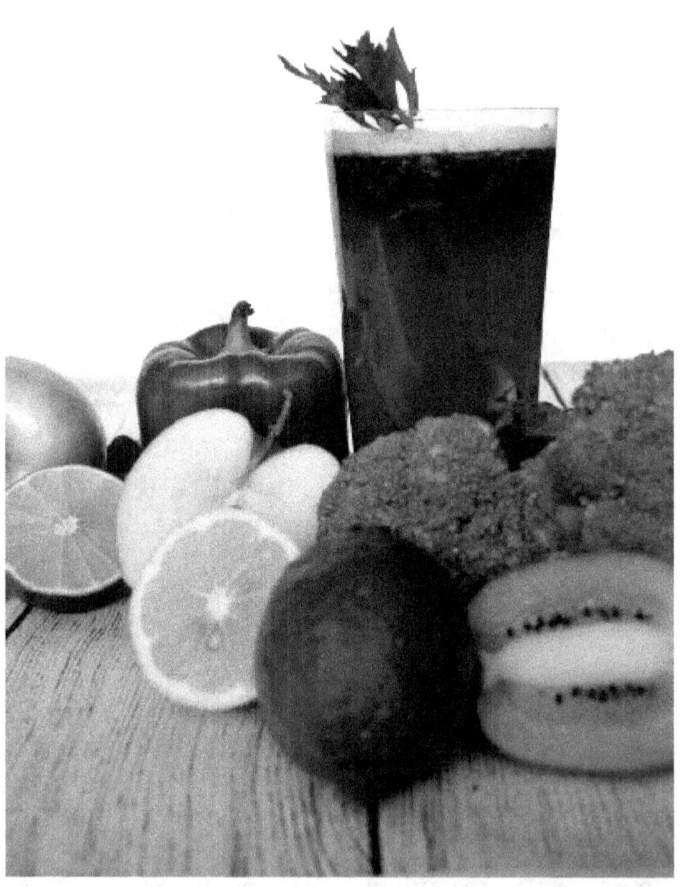

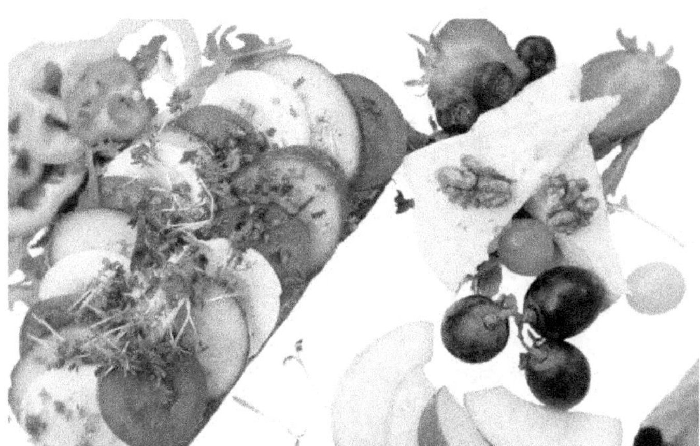